# Handbook for Epstein-Barr Virus

*Testing and Treatment In Severe, Chronic Pain Conditions*

Forest Tennant

(DrPH, MPH, MD)

Published by the
Tennant Foundation
West Covina, California

ISBN:9781955934459
LCCN:2024926413

<u>SPONSORS OF THIS BOOK</u>

Tennant Foundation
336-338 S. Glendora Ave.
West Covina, CA 91790-3043
Ph: 626-716-2689
Fax: 626-919-7497
Email: tennantfoundation92@gmail.com

All proceeds from the sale of this book will go to the Medical Study and Education Projects sponsored by the Tennant Foundation

336-338 S. Glendora Ave.
West Covina, CA 91790-3043
Ph: 626-716-2689
Fax: 626-919-7497
Email: tennantfoundation92@gmail.com

Special discounts are available on quantity purchases by corporations, associations, educators, and others. For details, contact one of the parties listed below.

U.S. trade bookstores and wholesalers: Please contact.

Nancy Kriskovich
Tel: (406)249-2002; or
email snkriskovich@gmail.com

# Disclaimer

The information in this handbook is only for educational purpose and advice to medically use it should come from a personal medical practitioner. Opinions and recommendations published here are neither sponsored nor approved by any party except the Tennant Foundation. Any recommendations in this handbook that are followed cannot guarantee clinical success or an absence of complications.


# Acknowledgements

Medical Director
Martin J. Porcelli, DO, MPHE, PhD

His anti-viral clinical care has permitted real life observations in chronic pain patients.

Acknowledgement
Ingrid Hollis

Her knowledge of infectious and chronic pain was essential in researching the material for this book.

Publication Development
Rebecca Cholcher-Marino
Nancy Kriskovich

# DEDICATION

Dr. Joseph Teitelbaum was the first physician to recognize and develop treatment approaches for viral-induced chronic pain conditions. His pioneering efforts as a sole practitioner with a scientific and entrepreneurial bent have been an inspiration for me to follow his work.

# Table of Contents


Authors Notes ... i

Prologue ... iii

Introduction ... 1

How EBV Reactivates and Causes Painful Disease ... 3

Stressful Events That Cause EBV Reactivation ... 8

Risk Factors for EBV Reactivation ... 10

Which Pain Patients Should Be Tested? ... 12

The Pathological Complications of EBV Reactivation ... 14

The Autoimmunity of EBV ... 17

Tissue Invasion and Infiltration ... 19

Key Test: Determination of Reactivation and Autoimmunity ... 21

How to Determine Current EBV Reactivation ... 24

The Most Common EBV Clinical Presentation: Interpretation and Actions Needed ... 26

Treatment of EBV Reactivation and Autoimmunity ... 29

Prevention of EBV Reactivation: Step One of Treatment ....30

Suppression of Autoimmunity and Inflammation ....34

Reduction of Viral Load ....41

Intravenous Infusions ....44

The Accompaniment of EBV and Other Viruses ....45

Summary ....47

Glossary of Terms used in This Book ....50

Selected Bibliography ....56

References ....58

Index ....64

# Authors Notes

The Epstein-Barr virus (EBV) is still regarded by many as a rather harmless virus that causes the "kissing disease." Indeed, this virus, like many others, may cause an initial resolvable infection and then become a dormant, harmless parasite in human tissues. EBV is now known, however, to be able, under certain circumstances, to reactivate, invade tissues, create an autoimmune state, and produce some severe painful conditions and cancers. EBV may develop its pathologic conditions in tandem with other viruses and bacteria such as Lyme or mycoplasma, but it is almost always a prime causative factor.

The pathologic process by which EBV causes severe chronic or intractable pain has now been clarified. Laboratory tests to determine EBV reactivation and autoimmunity have been developed and are available through local laboratories. I recommend that every person with a severe chronic pain condition that has lasted over 90 days and requires daily medication for relief be tested for EBV reactivation and autoimmunity.

Prevention and treatment measures, albeit early and preliminary, are available to every medical practitioner.

This handbook summarizes and makes recommendations on what is known to date. I began to earnestly study the relationship between viruses and intractable pain over two decades ago. In the past three years, I have reviewed well over 200 cases of severe chronic pain who have been tested for EBV.

What I have learned, I am passing on in this handbook. My mission in writing this handbook is that we now have some exciting and effective tools to begin treating the underlying cause of pain in addition to our current symptomatic and palliative treatments. My motivation is that I firmly believe that EBV reactivation and autoimmunity is a terrible disease that can progressively cause pathologic pain and degeneration to the point of gross debilitation, a bed-bound state, and premature death.

# Prologue

This handbook is a practical "How To" guide to assist medical practitioners in the testing and treatment of EBV reactivation and autoimmunity. A menu of laboratory tests is now available so practitioners can properly evaluate each patient's EBV status. EBV reactivation and autoimmunity is similar to diabetes, hyperlipidemia, renal disease, and some other medical conditions in that it may be asymptomatic and deleterious for a considerable time period before symptoms appear. Prevention of EBV reactivation is relatively simple, but the control of EBV autoimmunity requires more complex medical treatment. At this early stage, the benefits of the current therapeutic measures for EBV, albeit imperfect and inconsistent, add a positive element to our symptomatic and palliative care of severe pain conditions.

# Introduction

The Epstein-Barr Virus (EBV) is now known to be the cause of many severe chronic painful conditions and cancers.[5,10,15,55] Persons with severe chronic pain that lasts for over ninety days and requires daily medication for relief should be tested for EBV reactivation and autoimmunity (hereafter EBV R&A). Reactivation in both clinical practice and in this Handbook means that the virus has reactivated in the past and may or may not be active in the present. EBV autoimmunity remains constant. If EBV R&A is present, medical measures should be taken to prevent further reactivation, suppress autoimmunity, and reduce viral load.

EBV was initially discovered in 1964 by two virologists, Epstein and Barr, in a cancer known as Burkitt's lymphoma.[10] In 1968, it was found to be the cause of infectious mononucleosis.[13] Since that time, EBV has been identified as a causative factor or catalyst in several autoimmune diseases, multiple sclerosis, some cancers, and many painful conditions including adhesive arachnoiditis (AA).[7,11,12,14,16,45,52]

EBV is not usually the sole cause of any painful condition. The virus only reactivates to cause pain and cancer during periods of stress and immunocompromise.[4,8,30,38] Also, it usually works in tandem with other viruses and some bacteria to cause autoimmunity and severe pain.

Prevention and treatment measures for EBV R&A are not substitutes for the essential, symptomatic, and palliative measures required for severe chronic pain. The intent of EBV testing and treatment is to treat the underlying cause of pain as an "add on" to standard pain care.

# How EBV Reactivates and Causes Painful Disease

EBV is a universal herpes virus (Type 4) that usually enters the human body during infancy. The virus is active upon entry into the respiratory system and may cause the "sniffles" or other short term, respiratory condition. If the virus doesn't enter the body during infancy, it often does in one's teenage or early adulthood years by causing infectious mononucleosis. After EBV's initial activation and entry into the body, it settles in the membranes of the nose and throat and/or in lymphocytes. At this point, the virus is inactive and proceeds to live a dormant (latent), parasitic, and harmless life.[43] Blood tests will show a low level of antibodies to the virus while in its normal, quiescent state. It will remain in its dormant, harmless stage unless the body's immune system is lowered and weakened by some biologic stress at which time it can reactivate, invade tissues, produce autoantibodies (hereafter called autoimmunity), and cause a painful disease or a cancer.[21,23,31,44]

Many herpes viruses including EBV are known to enter the body, live a parasitic life, and reactivate under stress. A well-known example is herpes simplex (Types I and II) which may periodically develop blisters on the lips or genitalia. Herpes zoster and shingles following chicken pox is another example. A key medical point relative to EBV, like herpes simplex, is that a person may undergo a number of reactivations over time. In the case of EBV, each reactivation may produce both tissue invasion by the virus and additional autoantibodies. Unfortunately, EBV autoimmunity may cause tissue destruction that is initially asymptomatic but will eventually produce a symptomatic painful disease or cancer.[32,35,46]

The painful conditions that may develop from EBV R&A are quite variable and include such conditions as a herniated disc, spinal fluid leak, cancer, or fibromyalgia. These conditions may occur suddenly without warning. Often the patient doesn't connect his/her painful condition to a stressful event that may have occurred many years prior to the onset of their painful condition.[8,24,38] In summary, EBV reactivation, autoimmunity, and tissue invasion and infiltration may silently and asymptomatically progress for a considerable time period before a painful condition becomes obvious. In the author's experience a high percentage of severe chronic pain patients also develop a cancer after the onset of pain.

Throughout this handbook the abbreviation EBV R&A will be used for reactivation and autoimmunity. It implies that reactivation has taken place and both autoantibody formulation and tissue invasion by the virus has occurred.

A summary Table is attached on how EBV autoimmunity and tissue invasion may cause a painful condition. It is also noted that the pain that results can range from mild to extremely severe.

| **Tissues Attacked+** | **Pathologic Consequences** | **Effect on Bioelectricity*** |
|---|---|---|
| Nerves, cauda equina, arachnoid, discs | Inflammation, erosion, degeneration | Conduction impaired |
| Nerves, cauda equina, arachnoid | Adhesions, fibrosis, scarring | Blocked, entrapped |
| Small nerve fibers, glial cells, receptors | Eliminated | Accumulation |

*Anything that interferes or impairs bioelectricity produces pain.

+Other tissues besides the ones listed in the Table can be attacked.

## SCHEMATA OF EBV R&A

EBV Enters the Body

↓

Dormant, Parasite

↓

Biologic Stress

↓

Immune Protection Diminishes

↓

Virus Reactivates

↓

Autoantibodies Form

↓

Virus Invades Tissue

↓

Painful Condition and/or Cancer

# Stressful Events That Cause EBV Reactivation

EBV R&A doesn't just happen. The dormant parasitic virus reactivates when a biologic stress is severe enough to alter cortisol, adrenalin, and insulin/glucagon activity.[8,24,38] In turn, these hormonal alterations lower natural immune protection which gives the virus an opportunity to reactivate. The term "opportunistic" is clearly a characteristic of EBV.

Some stresses that can reactivate EBV have been identified. The most common stresses are trauma, infections, and psychologic.[8,24,38] Traumatic events include accidents, domestic violence, sports injuries, and invasive medical procedures such as surgery or epidural injections. Infections include Lyme, mycoplasma, meningitis, and infectious mononucleosis. Psychologic tribulations such as post-traumatic stress disorder (PTSD), divorce, death of a loved one, and bankruptcy may also cause hormonal alterations and an immunocompromised state.

The stressful event(s) that caused the first EBV reactivation may have occurred months or years before a painful condition develops. EBV reactivation can occur multiple times over a lifetime. With each reactivation protective antibodies as well as autoantibodies are created. Tissue invasion and infiltration may occur with each reactivation. Laboratory testing in cases of current and past reactivations will show high levels of antibodies to the viral capsid (capsule) antigen (hereafter VCA) and nuclear antigen (hereafter EBNA). The initials VCA and EBNA are used routinely on laboratory reports to identify the two major antibodies produced by EBV, and these abbreviations are used throughout this handbook.

TABLE

SOME STRESSFUL EVENTS WHICH CAN CAUSE EBV REACTIVATION

Trauma/accident
Invasive medical procedures
Severe infection
Psychologic tribulation
Nutritional deficiency
Sleep deprivation

# Risk Factors for EBV Reactivation

There are some risk factors or medical disorders that predispose or make a person more prone to EBV reactivation. A person with a risk factor plus a stressful event is a strong candidate for EBV R&A.

Any condition including some genetic diseases that weaken or compromise the natural immune system is a risk factor. Some medical conditions make tissues more susceptible to EBV invasion and infiltration due to defective tissue. For example, persons with a connective tissue or collagen disorder such as Ehlers-Danlos and/or Marfan syndromes, and osteogenesis imperfecta have well-known tissue deficiencies.

## TABLE

### SOME MEDICAL DISORDERS THAT ARE RISK FACTORS FOR EBV R&A

1. Genetic connective tissue/collagen disorders (e.g., Ehlers-Danlos, Marfan, others)
2. Genetic, anatomic structural defects (e.g., dwarfism, scoliosis, osteogenesis imperfecta)
3. Autoimmune disease (e.g., rheumatoid arthritis, psoriasis, ankylosing spondylitis, Crohn's disease)
4. Chronic medical diseases (e.g., diabetes, renal failure, cirrhosis, emphysema)

# Which Pain Patients Should Be Tested?

Any person who has had daily pain for over 90 days that is severe enough to require regular pain relief medication should be screened for EBV R&A. Persons who have chronic pain in more than one anatomic site (i.e., muscles, joints, head and spine, etc.) should be especially suspect. Some pain patients report "pain all over" which is usually a result of autoimmunity and small fiber neuropathy. Often, the person with EBV R&A will report that they have had pain that migrated from one anatomic site to another.

EBV causes painful conditions by direct tissue invasion and infiltration by the virus and by autoantibodies that attack and cause tissue destruction. Both the virus and its autoantibodies are carried to tissues by the blood stream, so pain can develop in multiple anatomic sites and migrate from one site to another. My blood test studies have identified some painful conditions which are usually associated with abnormal EBV R&A. Some are listed in the attached Table.

## TABLE

## CHRONIC PAINFUL CONDITIONS OFTEN ASSOCIATED WITH HIGH EBV VCA AND EBNA ANTIBODIES

| |
| --- |
| Adhesive arachnoiditis |
| Burning mouth/feet |
| Carpal tunnel syndrome |
| Fibromyalgia |
| Headache (constant, non-migraine) |
| Encephalomyelitis |
| Herniated discs (non-trauma, cervical and lumbar) |
| Pudendal neuropathy |
| Myofascial syndrome |
| Complex regional pain syndrome |
| Sciatica |
| Small fiber neuropathy |
| Tarlov cysts |

## The Pathological Complications of EBV Reactivation

When the immune system weakens due to a stressful event and allows EBV the opportunity to reactivate, two main pathologic effects are created that are responsible for developing a severe chronic pain condition. First, lymphocytes may carry the activated, replicating virus to tissues throughout the body. Once the lymphocyte is inside tissues ranging from glial cells in the brain to fascia around muscles, the lymphocyte may rupture and allow the activated virus to infiltrate and propagate in the tissues.[19,20] The invasion and infiltration of tissues may result in tissue inflammation followed by adhesions, fibrosis, and severe pain.[3,17] For unclear reasons EBV tissue infiltration may sometimes cause cancer. In the CNS the virus may cause demyelination of nerves.[5] Some tissues, which clinically and epidemiologically appear prone to invasion and infiltration, are lymph nodes, membranes, fascia, brain and spinal cord.[18-20,29,39,47] For example, EBV is highly associated with lymphoma and Hodgkin's disease, fibromyalgia, and the spinal disorders of multiple sclerosis and adhesive arachnoiditis. Glial cells in the CNS are a favorite EBV target.[19,20]

The second major pathologic effect of EBV reactivation is the development of autoantibodies.[31,32,40] When EBV reactivates, two protective antibodies, VCA and EBNA, are formed. Unfortunately, autoantibodies are also formed by multiple biologic mechanisms.[16,31,32] The EBV autoantibodies are like other autoantibodies in that they mistake normal tissues for some foreign organism or element. They, therefore, attack normal tissue causing inflammation, degeneration, scarring, and pain. Some favorite targets from a clinical perspective appear to be intervertebral discs, spinal canal membranes (i.e., arachnoid), and small nerve fibers.[55] Some EBV autoantibodies are carried on the EBNA antibody. Consequently, a blood test that shows a very high EBNA level can be assumed to carry autoantibodies that are tissue destructive and can cause a painful, clinical condition or cancer.

The two pathologic complications of EBV R&A may produce a plethora of medical disorders. In the clinical setting these cases may be considered "complex" and/or "untreatable." Indeed, they may manifest with a variety of symptoms besides pain.

## TABLE

## MAJOR PATHOLOGIC COMPLICATIONS OF EBV REACTIVAION

- ✓ Tissue invasion and infiltration
- ✓ Autoantibodies

Both complications may cause tissue inflammation, degeneration, scarring, and severe pain.

# The Autoimmunity of EBV

Autoimmunity occurs when autoantibodies are formed that attack one's own tissues. It is generally believed that the autoantibodies somehow mistake normal tissues to be a foreign organism or element.[45]

Some diseases have autoantibodies that can be identified by laboratory testing. The best known is probably the rheumatoid factor. The antinuclear autoantibody (ANA) is a "general" autoantibody that may develop in several autoimmune disorders including EBV autoimmunity.

EBV autoantibodies have been known to develop since 1974.[46] Various research studies show that EBV may create autoantibodies by multiple biologic mechanisms.[31,32] No specific laboratory test for EBV autoantibodies is yet available, but research is being done to develop a test.

Every EBV reactivation likely produces some autoantibodies. They are, therefore, cumulative over time. Some autoantibodies are carried on the EBNA antibody complex. Others simply may develop at the tissue level without entering the bloodstream. From a purely clinical perspective, an elevated EBNA antibody at least two times the upper normal laboratory level in a severe chronic pain patient, can be presumed to carry some autoantibodies that will continually attack tissues. Once tissue is attacked, inflammation, adhesions, fibrosis, and pain may ensue. EBV R&A may sometimes be associated with abnormal blood lymphocyte counts, and serum protein patterns. A positive ANA (antinuclear autoantibody) and elevated serum inflammatory markers, including interleukins, are common.[17]

> As noted in a later chapter, Step One of EBV treatment is to initiate some of the medicinals that laboratory studies have shown to prevent reactivation. Unfortunately, EBV autoantibodies, like those in rheumatoid arthritis and systemic lupus erythematosus, may never totally be eliminated or evacuated from the human body. While future or additional reactivations of EBV can usually be prevented, EBV autoimmunity will remain and require indefinite suppression by medical means.

# Tissue Invasion and Infiltration

When EBV reactivates, it is carried by lymphocytes into all body tissues including the brain and spinal cord. Once invasion occurs, EBV may replicate enough to break out of lymphocytes and take up residence in tissue. It seems to have a predilection for soft friable tissues such as small nerve fibers, fascia, disc centers, and membranes such as the arachnoid. Invasion may contribute to central pain as it may invade glial and other cells in the CNS.[18-20,39,55] Once it infiltrates tissue, it may cause inflammation, adhesions, fibrosis, and severe chronic pain. For unclear reasons, EBV may sometimes cause tissue to proliferate. This appears to be the mechanism for tumors and cancers. It also may be the cause of ligament and membrane hypertrophy intrinsic to such conditions as carpal tunnel syndrome and pudendal nerve entrapment.

Currently, there is no way to specifically determine if tissue invasion and infiltration has occurred. To definitely accomplish this, a biopsy, tissue culture, and/or imaging technique would be necessary, and these diagnostic tools are not yet available. Due to this limitation, the medical practitioner has to assume this development. For example, a patient with long-standing severe chronic pain and extremely high VCA and EBNA antibody levels can be presumed to have some EBV tissue invasion and infiltration.

# Key Test: Determination of Reactivation and Autoimmunity

In severe chronic pain conditions, the key clinical question is whether there is EBV R&A. This is indicated by high blood levels of VCA and EBNA. I suggest that the blood levels of these two antibodies be at least two times the upper, normal limits of the testing laboratory to assume that autoimmunity is present. Also, the patient must have a severe chronic pain condition to reasonably link high VCA and EBNA levels to the condition.

In summary, extremely high VCA and EBNA levels in a severe chronic pain patient can be reasonably assumed that both tissue invasion and infiltration by the virus and the development of autoantibodies have, over time, occurred and helped cause the painful condition.[16,20,29,31,42,45,51]

The renowned research laboratories known as ARUP (Association of Regional University Pathologists) in Salt Lake City, Utah have developed the test levels of VCA and EBNA antibodies that are currently used by most major laboratories. Attached is a Table showing the upper ARUP reference levels for VCA and EBNA antibodies. The two times normal levels are also given.

| ANTIBODY LEVELS FOR PRESUMPTION OF REACTIVATION AND AUTOIMMUNITY IN A SEVERE CHRONIC PAIN PATIENT | | |
|---|---|---|
| IgG Antibody | Reference Level | Minimal Level for R&A Presumption |
| VCA (viral capsid antigen) | 21.9 units/ml | 65.7 units/ml |
| EBNA (nuclear antigen) | 21.9 units/ml | 65.7 units/ml |

- ✓ Levels that are two or more times the upper reference levels can be assumed to represent recurrent reactivations in the past and the presence of autoimmunity if the patient also has a severe chronic pain condition.

- ✓ IgM antibodies that are elevated indicate a currently active infection, usually infectious mononucleosis. The IgM VCA is almost always negative in chronic pain patients.

- ✓ The maximal laboratory capability or limit for testing of VCA and EBNA antibodies is usually about 600-750 units per ml. If levels are above the maximal test level, it can be reasonably assumed that there has been multiple reactivations, and that autoimmunity and tissue infiltration is present.

# How to Determine Current EBV Reactivation

It is critical to determine if a person with severe chronic pain has current EBV reactivation as well as whether reactivation has occurred in the past. EBV can reactivate many times over a lifetime.[24,32,36,45,52] With each reactivation, additional autoantibodies and tissue invasion and infiltration will likely occur. If current reactivation is determined to be present, medical measures intended to reduce the body's viral load are warranted. Antiviral and anti-parasitic agents must be considered which are detailed in a later chapter.

Two blood tests have been recently developed to determine current reactivation:

1) Early Epstein-Barr nuclear antigen antibody – (Early EBNA IgG) (ARUP upper level is 11.0 units/ml)

2) Polymerase Chain Reaction (PCR) (normal is zero copies or units per ml)

A positive PCR test (or other DNA blood test) indicates that the virus is in the bloodstream and being transported to tissues. Repeat testing of early EBNA and/or PCR should be done to help determine if treatment is effective. Be clearly informed: the blood levels of VCA and EBNA do not usually reduce with treatment since they are protective antibodies that will remain for life.

> Testing Note: Even if EBV is not currently in a reactive state, autoimmunity will persist and require medical treatment.

# The Most Common EBV Clinical Presentation: Interpretation and Actions Needed

Presentation:

The most common clinical presentation is a patient who has a severe chronic pain condition that requires daily medication for pain relief and high elevations of both VCA and EBNA. Both antibody levels will be more than two times the upper normal laboratory level. Some levels may exceed laboratory testing capability (i.e., over 600 or 750 units per ml). The test for infectious mononucleosis which is the IgM VCA will be negative.

Interpretation

High elevations that are two times normal of both VCA and EBNA in a severe chronic pain patient indicates that EBV reactivation has occurred in the past and/or present and that autoimmunity is present and active.

## Prudent Actions to Be Taken

The first step, which is described in a later chapter, is to initiate some medicinals that will prevent further reactivation.

Medical measures to suppress EBV autoimmunity, as described in a later chapter, should be initiated. An early EBNA or PCR test should also be done to determine if there is current reactivation. If so, antiviral and/or anti-parasitic therapy is recommended.

## SUMMARY TABLE

### MOST COMMON CLINICAL PRESENTATION

1. Patient with severe chronic pain over 90 days that requires daily pain relief medication.

2. Blood test shows VCA and EBNA antibody elevations to be two or more times the upper normal limit for the testing laboratory.

3. The IgM VCA for infectious mononucleosis will be negative.

4. EBV R&A is present and medical therapy to prevent further reactivation and suppress autoimmunity and inflammation should be initiated.

# Treatment of EBV Reactivation and Autoimmunity

Treatment of EBV R&A falls into three categories:

1) Prevention of reactivation
2) Suppression of autoimmunity and inflammation
3) Reduction of viral load

A person with severe chronic pain and high elevations of VCA and EBNA will require combination treatment to prevent further reactivation and to suppress autoimmunity and inflammation. Prevention of reactivation is Step One because this step will hopefully halt further development of autoantibodies and tissue infiltration. If further reactivation is stopped, blood and tissue infiltration will eventually cease as the virus will die off. If there is current reactivation of EBV as indicated by an elevated early EBNA and/or PCR test, a reduction in viral load by anti-viral and/or anti-parasitic drugs should be attempted.

# Prevention of EBV Reactivation: Step One of Treatment

Some innovative researchers have tested a number of medicinals in laboratory settings to determine which ones prevent EBV reactivation. Some other medicinals have become popular with medical practitioners although no systematic studies and reports have yet been published on their ability to prevent reactivation.

Prevention of reactivation is "Step One" of EBV treatment because each reactivation produces additional autoantibodies and tissue invasion. If further reactivation is halted, EBV in tissues and blood will eventually die off. Unfortunately, EBV autoantibodies may be permanent as in the case of rheumatoid arthritis and other autoimmune diseases. Consequently, they cannot be totally eliminated by current medical measures; only suppressed.

The attached Table lists most of the agents identified in laboratory settings which prevent EBV reactivation. At this time, medical practitioners are using a variety of these medicinals based on personal choice. Many of the preventive medicinals have been put into combinations which are commercially available. The author's favorite prevention regimen is given here although it admittedly may not be the best:

- Vitamin C – 2000 mg in AM and PM
- Selenium – 100-200 mg a day
- Vitamin D (especially D-3)
- Vitamin B-12
- Curcumin

Besides the inhibitors listed in the Table, Monolaurin™, a coconut oil derivative, and some homeopathic formulations have become popular agents among many medical practitioners. To date, there are no systematic or controlled clinical studies that demonstrate serum reduction of early EBNA or PCR levels. Practitioners will have to review the available choices and choose the ones they prefer. Treatment effectiveness must be judged clinically on whether the patient reduces pain and other troublesome symptoms.

| TABLE<br>MEDICINALS FOR PREVENTION<br><br>OF EPSTEIN-BARR VIRUS REACTIVATION | |
|---|---|
| Vitamin C | Astragalus |
| Vitamin D | Curcumin |
| Resveratrol | Andrographis |
| Luteolin | Cimetidine |
| Selenium | Lysine |
| Zinc | |

The medicinals listed here have been shown in laboratory testing to have inhibitory activity on EBV reactivation.

## References

1. Andre G, Trompet E, Snoeck R. Novel therapeutics for Epstein-Barr virus. *Molecules* 2019;24:997-1009.
2. Eladwy RA, Vu HT, Shah R, et al. The fight against the carcinogenic Epstein-Barr virus: gut microbiota, natural medicines and beyond. *Int J Mol Sci* 2023;24:1716-1725.

3. Kerr J. Epstein-Barr virus (EBV) reactivation and therapeutic inhibitors. *J Clin Pathol* 2019;0:1-8.

# Suppression of Autoimmunity and Inflammation

EBV autoimmunity is one of the pathologic complications of EBV reactivation that causes severe chronic pain. Autoantibodies attack multiple tissues including membranes, fascia, small nerve fibers, cartilage, and even the glial cells in the CNS. EBV autoimmunity initially causes inflammation which proceeds to adhesions, fibrosis, tissue destruction, and severe pain. The main purpose of suppressing EBV autoimmunity and inflammation is to preserve tissues that have already been attacked as well as prevent additional tissues from being attacked. Unfortunately, it may not be possible to totally eliminate or "cure" EBV autoimmunity just as it has not been possible to totally eliminate or cure the autoimmunity of rheumatoid arthritis, psoriasis, or Sjogren's Syndrome. The goal, therefore, is to suppress and control EBV autoimmunity and inflammation. Three treatment approaches are being used to suppress autoimmunity and inflammation:[2]

1. Corticosteroids and anti-inflammatory agents.
2. Autoimmune suppressing agents.
3. Medicinals and nutrients to enhance immunity and tissue resistance.

Medical practitioners have a number of choices among the three approaches. Most are relatively new and have little clinical evaluation, but all have early, positive clinical reports from medical practitioners. Here is a summary of each.

Corticosteroids and Anti-inflammatory Agents:
This author strongly advocates combined use of a corticosteroid and an anti-inflammatory agent in a person with severe chronic pain and EBV R&A. Short term, high dose corticosteroids are often used for acute infectious mononucleosis, but EBV autoimmunity requires long-term use. I recommend low dose, intermittent use of corticosteroids to suppress and avoid the well-known side effects of corticosteroids (i.e., osteoporosis, pituitary dysfunction, hyperglycemia, etc.). Methylprednisolone or dexamethasone are the corticosteroids that have potent effects inside the CNS, so they are preferred if the pain patient has a CNS disorder like arachnoiditis or glial cell inflammation.[25,37,48,53] Typically, glial cell inflammation is associated with constant pain and possibly some hyperalgesia. If the pain involves only organs and tissue outside the CNS, prednisone and hydrocortisone may be superior agents.

This Table shows starting oral corticosteroid regimens.

TABLE

LOW DOSE, INTERMITTENT, ORAL CORTICOSTEROIDS

Methylprednisolone, 2 to 4 mg
Dexamethasone, 0.5 to 0.75 mg
Prednisone, 5 to 10 mg
Hydrocortisone, 10 to 20 mg

The above doses are administered 1 to 3 times a week.

Alternatives to oral corticosteroids include a weekly or bi-monthly corticosteroid injection. I highly recommend that persons with EBV R&A and severe chronic pain attend their practitioner's office for periodic injections. The reason being that the injection will be done efficiently, and the patient obtains psychologic and motivational support as the combination of severe chronic pain and EBV R&A is a very serious and debilitating disorder.

EBV R&A generated inflammation usually responds well to ketorolac (Toradol®).[28,40,42] Like corticosteroids, ketorolac is administered on a low dose, intermittent basis to maintain effectiveness while avoiding the side effects of gastrointestinal bleeding and renal impairment. A safe regimen is 10 to 30 mg taken one to two times a week by either the oral or injection routes. Even a dose as seldom as once or twice a month can be used. Ketorolac is both an analgesic and anti-inflammatory agent. Its unique effectiveness is partially related to its ability to cross the blood brain barrier and interact with N-methyl-d-aspartate receptors.[40]

Another anti-inflammatory agent that crosses the blood brain barrier and enters spinal fluid is diclofenac. It is a ketorolac alternative. Older anti-inflammatory agents may still be effective in some patients if the anatomical pain sites are outside the CNS. These agents include aspirin, ibuprofen, and naprosyn. Herbal and natural anti-inflammatory agents are worthy adjuncts to ketorolac and diclofenac.

I recommend the use of low dose naltrexone for pain control unless the patient is on daily opioids. Patients with severe chronic pain who are on opioids should remain on them as well as other medicinals that control pain. Like ketorolac, naltrexone has both analgesic and anti-inflammatory properties. My recommended starting dose is 0.5 to 1.0 mg given twice a day. The dose can be raised over time to as high as 14.0 mg a day given either as a single or divided dosage. A natural substance called palmitoylethanolamide (abbreviated PEA) also has both analgesic and anti-inflammatory properties. It can be used as either a flare or maintenance medication. Commercially, PEA has been combined with luteolin and this combination has become very popular with severe chronic pain patients who have EBV R&A. Luteolin is one of the agents shown in laboratory studies to prevent EBV reactivation.

## Autoimmune Suppressing Agents

Although early in clinical experience and evaluation, the long-standing autoimmune agents methotrexate and chloroquine are now being used for EBV R&A.[26] Dosages are low and intermittently used as is the case with corticosteroids and ketorolac. This author has received many anecdotal, positive reports on the use of methotrexate in EBV R&A, so its use is encouraged. Usual dosages of methotrexate range from 2.5 to 10 mg on a once or twice a week basis. Chloroquine has traditionally been used as both an autoimmune suppressor and anti-parasitic. It has not yet been used as much as methotrexate. It is detailed in the next chapter.

## Medicinals and Nutrients to Enhance Immunity and Tissue Resistance

The newest medical innovations to treat EBV R&A are medicinals and nutrients to enhance one's own immunity and tissue resistance. Tissue resistance is a new concept. Its rationale is that EBV cannot invade and infiltrate tissues that are strong, tight, and healthy. This concept is especially applicable to persons with genetic connective tissue/collagen deficiency disorders such as Ehlers-Danlos Syndrome. Several herbs, peptides, and hormones are becoming popular among patients with EBV R&A who have severe chronic pain. Examples of herbs are andrographis, curcumin, and serrapeptase. A popular peptide is thymosin. Other peptides have commercial names such as BPC-157 (Body Protection Compound) and KPV (lysine, proline, valine).

Adequate hormone levels are essential for both strong immunity and tissue resistance. Some composite, multiple hormones, especially colostrum and deer antler velvet, are being attempted. A group of hormones produced in the CNS called neurosteroids have been shown in laboratory studies to reduce pain and heal tissues.[6,22,38,50] The most popular is dehydroepiandrosterone (DHEA).[6,22] Severe chronic pain will depress hormone levels of testosterone, progesterone, estradiol, and pregnenolone.[50] All these hormones help sustain an effective immune system and aid in healing damaged tissue.[50] Blood testing and replacement of any deficient hormone is highly recommended.[22,34,50]

It is prudent to recommend a diet of adequate protein and low carbohydrate intake along with plentiful vegetables and fruits that may have anti-inflammatory properties (i.e., broccoli, apples, blueberries, etc.). Many patients with severe chronic pain shun or dislike protein foods such as fish, beef, and poultry. I usually recommend a collagen or amino acid supplement as I rarely find a patient with severe chronic pain who eats daily protein in adequate amounts.

Although there are various measures that have recently emerged to enhance the immune system, suppress autoimmunity, and build tissue resistance, they have not yet had much clinical experience. All lack the benefit of systematic or controlled study. They have solid, theoretical rationale for their use and medical practitioners are adopting them. Some measures may eventually become first line therapy. Medical practitioners may wish to attempt one or more of these measures and share their experiences.

# Reduction of Viral Load

When EBV reactivates the virus enters both blood and tissues. It accumulates in tissues through replication. At this time, the body load of active virus is assessed by the quantitative blood level of early EBNA antibodies and/or by PCR which measures EBV DNA in the blood. Elevations of either test calls for serious consideration of anti-viral and anti-parasitic agents.

Therapeutic trials of one or more of the standard antiviral agents are warranted to reduce viral presence in blood and tissue. They are shown in the Table with standard starting dosages.

| TABLE |
|---|
| STANDARD ANTIVIRAL AGENTS |
| Acyclovir (Zovirax®, 400 to 1000 mg a day) |
| Valacyclovir (Valtrex®, 500 to 1000 mg a day) |
| Famciclovir (Famvir® 500 to 1000 mg a day) |

Some physicians are combining standard agents and/or varying standard dosages. Also, low dose, long-term maintenance is now used to suppress EBV R&A. Examples are acyclovir 200 mg a day or valacyclovir 500 mg on three days a week.

The antiviral agents have been inconsistent in both converting early EBNA and PCR tests to normal as well as reducing pain and other symptoms. Consequently, two anti-parasitic drugs are now being attempted. The most popular agent is ivermectin (Stromectol®). Dosages range widely among practitioners. I recommend a dosage of about 6 to 9 mg a day for five to seven days followed by 3 to 6 mg on one or two days a week. Besides viral load reduction, ivermectin may also have some direct anti-inflammatory properties.

Chloroquine, an anti-malarial drug is now being attempted. The daily dose is 250 to 500 mg. A trial of a few weeks is a reasonable approach to reduce viral load.

Anecdotal reports suggest that the combination of anti-viral or anti-parasite drugs are more effective when used with corticosteroids and anti-inflammatory agents such as ketorolac. For example, a controlled study with famciclovir and celecoxib directed at herpes simplex and fibromyalgia was quite effective.

It should be noted that antiviral or anti-parasite treatment will not usually lower blood levels of VCA and EBNA antibodies. These antibodies have been developed by the body for lifetime protection. Successful reduction of the body's viral load, however, can be documented by lowering early EBNA or PCR blood levels.

# Intravenous Infusions

Two intravenous infusions are being used to treat EBV. I have received many positive reports on both:

1. Vitamin C
2. Methylprednisolone

The dosage of these two infusions has been quite variable. They have been given on a one-time basis or for two to five continuous days. Vitamin C infusions have each ranged from about 5000 to 15,000 mg. Methylprednisolone has ranged from about 50 to 500 mg.

Both of these infusions usually result in a significant reduction in pain and an increase in energy and feeling of well-being. These positive outcomes may last up to about three months. They may not be curative, but they give the patient a great reprieve from their misery and a window to put together a better, quality life. I know of no permanent side effects from these infusions. Infusions also give the medical practitioner and patient some time to "get to know" one another. They are highly recommended as an adjunct to an ongoing medical program.

# The Accompaniment of EBV and Other Viruses

EBV R&A is almost always accompanied by high antibody levels of other viruses. Antibodies to the bacteria, Lyme and mycoplasma, may occasionally accompany EBV.

The clinical significance of multiple, elevated viral antibody levels is unclear. It is likely that there is a synergistic effect between EBV and other viruses. For example, the prestigious and pioneering Immuno Sciences Laboratory in Los Angeles, California has found that the combination of EBV, herpes virus Type 6, and SARS-Covid-2 is a potent autoimmune triad.

In my viral test reviews of well over 200 persons with severe chronic pain, every patient with elevated VCA and EBNA also demonstrated an elevation of antibodies to one or more other viruses. Elevated viral antibody levels other than EBV that I have encountered are listed in the attached Table. There has been no consistent pattern.

In a study of 110 cases of adhesive arachnoiditis I found only three cases that did not have elevated EBV antibodies. All three are males who developed severe pain before the age of thirty. All three had high antibody levels of multiple viruses, except EBV. My only possible explanation is that another virus invaded and/or reactivated in the early life of these individuals and this virus(s) somehow prohibited EBV from ever reactivating.

It may be appropriate to use the label, multi-virus reactivation and autoimmunity rather than EBV R&A. If a severe chronic pain patient has high antibody levels to multiple viruses, including EBV, some consideration must be given that the patient has significant immune deficiency and requires potent and long-term treatment.

TABLE

ELEVATED VIRAL ANTIBODIES FOUND IN PATIENTS WITH EBV REACTIVATION AND SEVERE CHRONIC PAIN

Coxsackie
SARS-Covid-2
Cytomegalovirus
Para-virus
Herpes I, II and VI
Rubella
Rubeola
Varicella
Mumps

# Summary

1. EBV can reactivate from a harmless, dormant parasitic state and cause some cancers and severe chronic pain conditions.

2. It is recommended that all persons who have had chronic pain for over ninety days and requires daily medication for relief should be tested for EBV R&A.

3. EBV may reactivate due to any severe biologic stress including trauma, infection, psychologic tribulation, invasive medical procedure, sleep deprivation, or nutritional deficiency.

4. When EBV reactivates it forms two major antibodies. One is to the virus capsid antigen antibody, abbreviated VCA, and the other is virus nuclear antigen antibody abbreviated EBNA.

5. EBV reactivation produces autoantibodies as well as tissue invasion and infiltration. Both pathologic developments may cause tissue inflammation, adhesions, fibrosis, and severe chronic pain.

6. EBV reactivation may produce severe chronic pain in multiple anatomic sites. EBV R&A has a

predilection for small nerve fibers, fascia, membranes, cartilage, and the central nervous system.

7. High levels of VCA and EBNA, at least two times normal, indicate the likely presence of autoimmunity and tissue invasion if the person also has severe chronic pain.

8. The first step in EBV treatment is to prevent further reactivation. Several medicinals including vitamins C and D, and the minerals selenium and zinc, and the herbals, curcumin, and luteolin, have been shown in laboratory testing to prevent reactivation.

9. EBV autoimmunity and inflammation requires medical treatment. Low dose, intermittent use of a corticosteroid and ketorolac (Toradol®) are preferentially recommended.

10. The EBV viral load, as indicated by early EBNA and/or PCR test, may be reduced by antiviral or anti-parasitic agents. Results to date, however, have been inconsistent.

11. The information presented here represents a new medical concept in disease formation. The understanding of EBV R&A, its complications, and

treatment will undoubtedly advance and improve over the messages and suggestions in this handbook.

12. EBV testing and treatment should now be added as a curative measure to the usual symptomatic and palliative care of severe chronic pain.

# Glossary of Terms used in This Book

Adhesive Arachnoiditis: An intraspinal canal inflammatory disorder in which a clump or mass of cauda equina nerves are glued by adhesions to the arachnoid-dural covering of the spinal canal.

Antibody: a substance produced by B lymphocytes in response to an offending antigen. There are five antibody classes known as immunoglobulins: IgA, IgD, IgE, IgG, and IgM. IgM is the earliest antibody produced against a virus but disappears from the serum after a short time period. IgG is the antibody produced by the body for long-term protection.

Arachnoiditis: Inflammation of the arachnoid layer of the spinal canal covering (meninges) without any nerves adhered to it. This condition cannot specifically be identified by MRI. It is a clinical diagnosis based on signs, symptoms, and laboratory tests.

Autoimmune Disease: A disease in which a person's own tissues are mistaken by an autoantibody or other element to be an outside invader such as a virus or bacteria and attacks and destroys one's own tissues.

Autoantibody: A globulin protein that attacks normal tissues to cause inflammation, tissue destruction, scarring, pain, and cancer.

Autoimmunity: An internal disease process that attacks and destroys tissue by an autoantibody.

Biologic Stress: A medical, nutritional, traumatic, or infectious event that causes extended adrenal and pancreatic hormonal alterations.

Cauda equina: About two dozen nerves that emanate from the spinal cord at the level of thoracic 12(T-12) or lumbar 1 (L-1) vertebrae and are suspended in spinal fluid. The term nerve roots is often applied rather than nerves.

Chronic Pain: A pain that persists longer than the usual healing time of about ninety days.

Collagen: A strong fibrous insoluble protein found in connective tissue including the dermis, tendons, ligaments, fascia, bone, cartilage, nerves, and membranes.

Connective Tissue Disorder: A genetic disease in which collagen in tissues is deficient and weakens the tissues which may result in inflammation, adhesions, scarring, and pain.

Corticoid or Corticosteroid: A pharmaceutical that is chemically related to cortisone.

Dormant: State in which a parasitic virus is in tissues but inactive and not causing any pathologic complications.

Ehlers-Danlos Syndrome (EDS): A genetic connective tissue disorder named after two physicians who first described the condition. The most common form is hypermobile.

Epstein-Barr Autoimmunity: An internal disease state in which EBV has reactivated and produced autoantibodies or equivalent process that causes tissue inflammation, destruction, pain, and cancer.

Epstein-Barr Nuclear Antigen Antibody (abbreviated EBNA): A protective antibody to the nucleus of the EBV which is formed with each reactivation. It increases in the blood with each reactivation and carries some autoantibodies.

Epstein Barr Virus: A virus of the herpes class (No. 4) that is normally an innocuous human parasite but may reactivate and produce an autoimmune disorder and a number of pathologic conditions including some cancers and painful diseases. Named after the scientists who discovered the virus in a cancer known as Burkitt's lymphoma.

Epstein Barr Virus: A virus of the herpes class (No. 4) that is normally an innocuous human parasite but may reactivate and produce an autoimmune disorder and a number of pathologic conditions including some cancers and painful diseases. Named after the scientists who discovered the virus in a cancer known as Burkitt's lymphoma.

Erosion: Tissue degeneration similar to rust of a metal.

Fibromyalgia: Diffuse pain in muscle groups and their fibrous connections to ligaments, fascia, and bone.

Fibrosis: The development of thickened and hardened tissue that may entrap nerves and blood vessels so that bioelectric conduction and blood flow are impaired.

Herb: A medicinal that comes from a plant or botanical.

Inflammation: Tissue that is red, hot, degenerating tissue followed by pain and functional impairment.

Immunocompromised: The immune system has weakened and is unable to ward off or eliminate infections.

Immunoglobulin-IgG: A protein antibody that is made by B lymphocytes and plasma cells that help the body fight infection.

Immunoglobulin-M: First antibody to appear when the body is exposed to an antigen. It disappears after a short time period.

Infiltration: The process of EBV spreading and multiplying in tissues.

Intractable Pain: Constant, incurable pain that may produce cardiovascular, respiratory, endocrine, and metabolic complications.

Invasion: The act that EBV has attached to or enters tissue.

In Vivo: Growth of tissue or a microbe in the body.

In Vitro: Growth of tissue or a microbe outside the body as in a test tube, plate, or dish.

Latent Phase: A state after initial infection when a virus is quiet, silent, and harmless. Same meaning as dormant.

Lymphocyte: A white blood cell which makes up about 25% of the body's total white blood cells. There are two main types: The B cell makes antibodies for immune protection and T cells that help B lymphocytes and/or remove cells that contain an offending infectious agent.

Lymphoma: A cancer of lymph tissues which may cause enlargement of lymph nodes.

Lytic Phase: Period in which a virus is multiplying or replicating by dividing itself.

Marfan Syndrome: A hereditary disorder of connective tissue, bones, muscles, ligaments, and skeletal structures. It is characterized by a tall lean body with long fingers, toes, joint flexibility, and flat feet.

Multi-Site, Migratory Pain Disease: Condition in which pain simultaneously occurs in multiple anatomic sites and the pains, overtime, will migrate to additional or different anatomical sites.

Natural: A medicinal that is made in the human body.

Opportunistic: The condition when one's natural immune system weakens and gives the virus the opportunity to reactivate from its dormant state.

Reactivation: A change from a dormant, carrier state to one in which the virus begins to duplicate and becomes an active infectious agent that can produce painful diseases and cancer.

Risk Factor: Any medical condition that weakens the immune system or natural tissue structure and gives EBV an opportunity to reactivate, invade, or infiltrate tissues.

Spinal canal: The spinal canal is a structure like a closed pipe that carries the spinal fluid. The fluid is primarily produced in the brain and flows down the canal on one side and flows back up to the brain to be diverted into lymph nodes and the general blood and lymphatic systems. The word canal is preferentially used here to simplify understanding.

Spine: Refers to the entire spine including vertebrae, intervertebral discs, spinal canal, cord inside the canal, and cauda equina nerves.

Viral Capsid Antigen Antibody (abbreviated VCA): Antibody of the IgG class that forms to the capsule (capsid) of the EBV. It is a protective antibody that increases in the serum with each viral reactivation.

# Selected Bibliography

1. Hoagland RJ. Infectious mononucleosis. Grune & Stratton, New York & London, 1967.
2. Jefferies, WM. Safe Uses of Cortisol. Charles C. Thomas Ltd, Springfield, Ill, 3rd ed, 2004.
3. Kines K. The Epstein-Barr Virus Solution. Coppell, TX, 2023.
4. Levy TE. Vitamin C, Infectious Diseases and Toxins: Curing the Incurable. Xlibris Corp, 2002.
5. Teitelbaum J. Pain Free 1-2-3. McGraw-Hill, New York, 2005.
6. Teitelbaum J. From Fatigue to Fantastic. Avery, New York, 2020, 4th ed.
7. Teitelbaum J. The Fatigue and fibromyalgia Solution. Avery, New York, 2013.
8. Teitelbaum J, Gottlieb B. Real Cause, Real Cure. Rondale, USA, 2011.
9. Tennant F. The Epstein-Barr Virus: A New Factor in the Care of Chronic Pain. Tennant Foundation, West Covina, CA, 2024.

10. William A. Medical Medium: Secrets Behind Chronic and Mystery Illness and How to Finally Heal. Hay House Inc., Carlsbad, CA, 2021.

11. Robertson ES. Epstein-Barr Virus. Caister Academic Press, Wymondham, England, 2005.

# References

1. Aalto SM, Linnavuori K, Peltola, et al. Immunocostivation of Epstein-Barr virus due to cytomegalovirus disease. *J Med Virol* 1998;56:186-91.Andre G, Trompet E, Snoeck R. Novel therapeutics for Epstein-Barr virus. *Molecules* 2019;24:997-1009.
2. Anderson D, Fanberge I, Hedstrom AK. Treatment options for Epstein-Barr virus related disorders of the central nervous system. *Infect and Drug Resist* 2023;16:4599-4620.
3. Bilello J, Tennant F. Patterns of chronic inflammation in extensively treated patients with arachnoiditis and chronic intractable pain. *Postgrad Med* 2016;92:1-5.
4. Binne UK, Amun W, Furrell PJ. Promotor sequence required for reactivation of Epstein-Barr virus from latency. *J Virology* 2002;76:10282-10289.
5. Bjornevik K, Cortese M, Healy BC, et al, et al. Longitudinal analysis reveals high prevalence of Epstein-Barr virus associated with multiple sclerosis. *Science* 2022;375:296-301.
6. Chang DM, Chu SJ, Chen HC, et al. Dehydroepiandrosterone suppresses interleukin 10 synthesis in women with systemic lupus erythematosus. *Ann Rheum Dis* 2004;63:1623-1620.
7. Cohen JL. Epstein-Barr Virus infection. *New Eng J* Med 2000;343:481-492.
8. Coskum O, Sener K, Kilic S, et al. Stress-related Epstein-Barr virus reactivation. *Clin Exp Med* 2010;10:15-20.
9. Duan Y, et al. Immune cell infiltration and the genes associated with ligamentum flavum hypertrophy:

identification and validation. *Front Cell Dev Biol* 2022;10:91478.

10. Epstein MA, Barr YM, Achang BC. Virus particles in cultured lymphocytes from Burkitt's lymphoma. Lancet 1964;1:702-703.
11. Harley JB, Chan X, Pujato M, et a. Transaction factors operate across disease loci, with EBNA2 implicated in autoimmunity. *Nat Genet* 2018;50:699-707.
12. Harrow T. Epstein-Barr virus could be a cause of multiple autoimmune disorders. *VA Research Currents* April 18, 2018.
13. Henle G, Henle N, Diehl V. Relation of Burkitt's tumor associated herpes type virus to infectious mononucleosis. *Proc Natl Acad* Sci 1968;59:94-101.
14. Henle G, Henle W, Klein G, et al. Antibodies to early Epstein-Barr virus-induced antigens in Burkitt's lymphoma. *J Nat Cancer Inst* 1971;46:861-871.
15. Henle W, Henle G. Epstein-Barr virus-related serology in Hodgkin's disease. *Nat Cancer Inst Monograph* 1973;36:79-84.
16. Houen G, Trier NH. Epstein-Barr virus and systemic autoimmune disease. *Front Immunol* 2020;11:1-13.
17. Hsu D, Malefytro W, Fiorentino DF, et al. Expression of interleukin-10 activity by Epstein-Barr virus protein BCRF 1. *Science* 1990;250:830-832.
18. Indari O, Tiwari D, Tanwar M, et al. Early biomolecular changes in brain microvascular endothelial cells under Epstein-Barr virus influence: A Raman microspectroscopic investigation. *Integr Biol* 2022;14:89-97.
19. Indari O, Jakhomola S, Pathak DK, et al. Comparative account of biomolecular changes post Epstein Barr virus infection of the neuronal and glial cells using Raman microspectroscopy. *ACS Chem Neurosci* 2022;13:1627-1637.

20. Jakhmola S, Jha HM. Glial cell response to Epstein Barr Virus infection: a plausible contribution to virus-associated inflammatory reactions in the brain. *Virology* 2021;559:182-195.
21. Jha HC, Pei Y, Robertson ES. Epstein-Barr virus: disease linked to infection and transformation. *Front Microbiol* 2016;7:1-16.
22. Jones KJ. Gonadal steroids and neuronal regeneration: a therapeutic role. *Adv Neurol* 1993;59:227-240.
23. Kenney SC, Mertz JE. Regulation of the latent-lytic switch in Epstein-Barr virus. *Semin Cancer Biol* 2014;26:60-68.
24. Kerr J. Epstein Barr Virus (EBV) reactivation and therapeutic inhibitors. *J Clin Pathol* 2019;0:1-8.
25. Kiefer R, Kreutzberg GW. Effects of dexamethasone on microglial activation in vitro. *J Neuroimmunology* 1991;34:99-108.
26. Kingsbury SR, Tharmanathan P, KKeding A, et al. Pain reduction with oral methotrexate in knee osteoarthritis. *Ann Intern Med* 2024;177:1145-1156.
27. Klanner FR. The treatment of poliomyelitis and other virus diseases with vitamin C. *So Med Surg* 1949;111:209-214.
28. Kumar K, Polston GR, Wallace MS. The effect of intravenous ketorolac on capsaicin-induced deep tissue hyperalgesia. *Anesth Analg* 2006;103:696-702.
29. Li YL, Wang JY, Lil K, et al. Epstein-Barr virus to be a trigger of autoimmune glial fibrillary acidic protein astrocytopathy. *CNS Neurosci Ther* 2023;29:4139-4146.
30. Libert N, Bigailon C, Chargari C, et al. Epstein-Barr virus reactivation in critically ill immunocompetent patients. *Biomed J* 2015;38:70-76.
31. Nagata K, Hayashi K. Epstein-Barr virus reactivation-induced immunoglobulin production: significance on autoimmunity. *Microorganisms* 2020;8:1875-1890.

32. Nakamura M, Burasteros F, Vaki Y, et al. Proving the normal and autoimmune B cell repertoire with Epstein-Barr virus, frequency of B cells producing monoreactive high affinity autoantibodies in patients with Hashimoto's disease and systemic lupus erythematosus. *J Immunnol* 1998;141:4165-4172.
33. Okano M, Kawa K, Kimura H, et al. Proposed guidelines for diagnosing chronic active Epstein-Barr infection. *Am J Hematol* 2005;80:64-69.
34. Reddy DS. Neurosteroids: endogenous role in the human brain and therapeutic potentials. *Prog Brain Res* 2010;186:13-137.
35. Rhodes G, Pumpold H, Kurki P, et al. Autoantibosies in infectious mononucleosis have specificity for the glycine-alanine repeating region of the Epstein-Barr virus nuclear antigen. *J Exp Med* ***1987;165:1026-1040.***
36. Rickinson AB. Chronic symptomatic Epstein-Barr virus infection. *Immunol Today* 1986;7:13-14.
37. Romundstad L, Breivik A, Niemi G, et al. Methylprednisolone intravenously 1 day after surgery has sustained analgesic and opioid-sparing effects. *Acta Anaesthesiol Scand* 2004;48:1223-1231.
38. Sausen DG, Bhutt o MS, Gallo ES, et al. Stress-induced Epstein-Barr virus reactivation. *Biomolecules* 2021;11:1380-1410.
39. Soni N, Ora R, Sing P, et al. Unpacking the CNS manifestations of Epstein-Barr virus: an imaging perspective. *Amer J Neurorad* 2023;44:1002-1008.
40. Sotgin ML, Riella G, Formaglio F, et al. Central effort of ketorolac involving NMDA receptors activity. *Brain Res* 1998;223-226
41. Strauss SE. The chronic mononucleosis syndrome. *J Infect Dis* 1988;157:405-412.

42. Stubhaug A, Romundstad L, Kaasa T, et al. Methylprednisolone and ketorolac rapidly reduce hyperalgesia around a skin burn injury and increase pressure pain thresholds. *Acta Anaesth Scand* 2007;51:1138-1146.
43. Sumaya CV, Henle W, Henle G, et al. Seroepidemiologic study of Epstein-Barr virus infections in a rural community. *J Infect Disease* 1975;131:403-408.
44. Sumaya, CV. Endogenous reactivation of Epstein-Barr virus infection. *J Infect Dis* 1977;135:374-379.
45. Sunderson B, Shirafkan F, Ripperger K, et al. The role of viral infections in the onset of autoimmune diseases. *Viruses* 2023;15:782-814.
46. Sutton RN, Emond RT, Thomas DB, et al. The occurrence of autoantibodies in infectious mononucleosis. *Clin Exp Immunol* 1974;17:427-436.
47. Takahashi H, Sugura T, Okazimo Y, et al. Inflammatory cytokines in the herniated disc of the lumbar spine. Spine 1996;21:218-224.
48. Takedo K, Sawamura S, Sekiyama H, et al. Effect of methylprednisolone on neuropathic pain and spinal glial activation in rats. *Anesthesiology* 2004;100:1249-1257.
49. Teitelbaum J. Effective treatment for chronic fatigue syndrome and fibromyalgia: an overview and 35 treatments for tough cases. *Townsend Letter* Nov, 2015:56-59.
50. Tennant F. The physiologic effects of pain on the endocrine system. *Pain* Ther 2013;2:75-86.
51. Tiwari D, Mittal N. Unraveling the links between neurodegeneration and Epstein-Barr virus-mediated cell cycle dysregulation. *Curr Res Neurobiol* 2023;3:2665-2945.
52. Vaughn JH. The Epstein-Barr virus in autoimmunity. *Springer Semin Immunopathol* 1995;17:203-230.

53. Werner MY, Lassen B, Kehlet H. Analgesic effects of dexamethasone in burn injury. *Reg Anesth Pain Med* 2002;27:254-260.
54. Zang Y, Chee A, Shi P, et al. Intervertebral disc cells produce interleukins found in patients with back pain. *Am J Phys Med* 2016;95:407-415.
55. Zhang N, Zou Y, Jiang L, et al. Epstein Barr virus and neurologic diseases. *Front Mol Biosci* 2022;10:1-34.

# Index

Activation, 3
Acyclovir, 42
Adhesions, 14, 18, 19, 34, 47, 50, 51
Adhesive arachnoiditis, 1, 14, 45
Adulthood, 3
Amino acid, 40
Andrographis, 39
Antibody, 15, 17, 20, 24, 26, 45, 46, 47, 50, 52, 53, 55
Antinuclear autoantibody, 17, 18
Arachnoiditis, 35, 50, 58
ARUP, 21
Association of Regional University Pathologists, 21
Autoimmunity, i, ii, iii, 1, 2, 3, 4, 12, 17, 21, 22, 23, 27, 29, 34, 35, 40, 46, 48, 59, 60, 62
Bankruptcy, 8
Biologic, 3, 8, 15, 17, 47
Body, 3, 14, 19, 24, 39, 41, 43, 50, 53, 54
Brain, 14, 19, 37, 55, 59, 60, 61
Cancer, 1, 3, 4, 14, 15, 50, 52, 54, 55
Cardiovascular, 53
Carpal tunnel, 19
Carrier, 55
Cauda equina, 50, 55
Causative, i, 1
Chloroquine, 38
Chronic pain, 5, 7, i, ii, 1, 2, 4, 12, 14, 17, 19, 20, 21, 22, 24, 26, 29, 34, 35, 36, 37, 38, 39, 40, 45, 46, 47, 48, 49
Clinical, 5, 15, 17, 21, 26, 31, 35, 38, 40, 45, 50
Collagen, 10, 39, 40, 51
Colostrum, 39

Complications, 15, 34, 51, 53
Connections, 53
Connective tissue, 10, 51, 54
Contain, 54
Control, iii, 34, 37
Controll, 31, 40, 42
Corticosteroids, 34, 35
Curcumin, 39, 48
Cytomegalovirus, 58
Death, 8
Deer antler velvet, 39
Deficiency, 39, 46, 47
Dehydroepiandrosterone, 39
Destruction, 4, 12, 34, 50, 52
Dexamethasone, 35, 60, 63
DHEA, 39
Diabetes, iii
Diagnosis, 50
Discs, 15, 55
Disease, iii, 1, 3, 4, 10, 14, 17, 30, 50, 51, 52, 55, 56, 58, 59, 60, 61, 62, 63
Disorder, 8, 10, 35, 36, 50, 52, 54
Divorce, 8
Dormant, i, 3, 8, 47, 54, 55
Dura, 50
Ehlers-Danlos, 39, 52, 71
Endocrine, 53, 62
Entrapment, 19
Epidural, 8
Epstein, 1
Epstein Barr, 52, 59, 60, 63
Factor, i, 1, 10, 17
Famciclovir, 42
Fibromyalgia, 4, 14, 42, 56, 62
Fibrosis, 18, 19, 34, 47
Genes, 58
Genetic, 10, 39, 51, 52
Genetic connective tissue, 39, 52
Glial cells, 14, 34, 35, 59
Guidelines, 61
Herniated disc, 4
Herpes, 3, 45, 52, 59
Herpes simplex, 3, 4, 42
Hormones, 39
Hydrocortisone, 35
Identified, 1, 8, 12, 17, 30, 50
Immune system, 3, 10, 14, 39, 40, 53, 55
Immuno Sciences Laboratory, 45
Impairment, 37, 53
Incurable, 53

Infancy, 3
Infiltration, 4, 9, 10, 12, 14, 19, 20, 21, 23, 24, 29, 47, 58
Inflammation, 14, 15, 18, 19, 29, 34, 35, 36, 47, 48, 50, 51, 52, 58
Injury, 62, 63
Interleukin, 18, 58, 59, 63
Intractable pain, i, ii, 58
Invasion, 4, 5, 9, 10, 12, 14, 19, 20, 21, 24, 30, 47, 48
Ivermectin, 42
Ketorolac, 36, 37, 38, 42, 48, 60, 61, 62
Kissing disease, i
Laboratory, iii, 9
Latent, 3, 60
Layer, 50
Leak, 4
Ligamentum flavum, 4
Luteolin, 38, 48
Lyme, i, 8, 45
Lymph nodes, 14, 54, 55
Lymphatic, 55
Lymphoma, 1, 14, 52, 59
Lysine, 39
Lytic, 54
Marfan Syndrome, 54
Mass, 50
Measures, i, iii, 1, 2, 24, 27, 30, 40
Medical, iii, 1, 4, 8, 10, 15, 19, 24, 30, 31, 35, 38, 40, 44, 47, 48, 51, 55
Membrane, 3, 14, 15, 19, 34, 48, 51
Meningitis, 8
Metabolic, 53
Methotrexate, 38, 60
Methylprednisolone, 35, 44, 61, 62
Migratory, 54
Misery, 44
Multiple sclerosis, 1, 14, 58
Multi-Site, 54
Muscle, 12, 14, 53, 54
Mycoplasma, i, 8, 45
Naltrexone, 37
Nerves, 14, 50, 51, 55
Neurologic, 63
Opioids, 37
Opportunistic, 8
Osteogenesis imperfecta, 10
Pain, iii, 1, 2, 4, 12, 14, 15, 18, 19, 26, 31, 34, 35, 37, 39, 42, 44, 46, 49, 50, 51, 52, 53, 54, 56, 60, 62, 63, 70, 72

Palliative, ii, iii, 2, 49
Palmitoylethanolamide, 37
Pancreatitis, 51
Parasite, 42, 52
Parasitic, 3, 8, 24, 27, 29, 38, 41, 42, 47, 48, 51
Pathologists, 21
Peptide, 39
Physician, 41, 52
Polymerase Chain Reaction, 24
Prednisone, 35
Pregnenolone, 39
Prevalence, 58
Prevention, i, iii, 2, 29, 30
Progesterone, 39
Proline, 39
Protein, 18, 39, 40, 50, 51, 53, 59, 60
Psoriasis, 34
PTSD, 8
Rationale, 38, 40
Reactivation, i, ii, iii, 1, 4, 8, 9, 10, 15, 17, 24, 27, 29, 30, 32, 33, 34, 38, 46, 47, 48, 52, 55, 58, 60, 61, 62
Regeneration, 60
Respiratory, 3, 53
Rheumatoid arthritis, 30, 34
Risk factors, 10
SARS-Covid, 45
Selenium, 48
Serrapeptase, 39
Shingles, 4
Sjogren's Syndrome, 34
Sleep, 47
Small fiber neuropathy, 12
Spinal canal, 15, 50, 55
Spinal fluid, 4, 37, 51, 55
Stage, iii, 3
Stress, 1, 3, 8, 47
Symptom, iii, 2, 4, 49, 61
Symptomatic, ii
Symptoms, iii, 15, 31, 42, 50
Teenage, 3
Testosterone, 39
Therapeutic, 41
Thymosin, 39
Tissue, 4, 5, 10, 12, 14, 15, 17, 18, 19, 20, 21, 23, 24, 29, 30, 34, 35, 39, 40, 41, 47, 48, 50, 51, 52, 53, 54, 55, 60
Toxins, 56
Trauma, 8, 47, 51

Treatment, 7, i, ii, iii, 2, 25, 29, 30, 34, 42, 46, 48, 49, 60, 62
Tumor, 19, 59
Valacyclovir, 42
Valine, 39
Viral load, 1, 24, 29, 42, 43, 48
Virologist, 1
Virus, i, ii, 1, 2, 3, 45, 46
Vitamin, 31, 32, 44, 56
Zinc, 48

<u>OTHER BOOKS BY FOREST TENNANT</u>

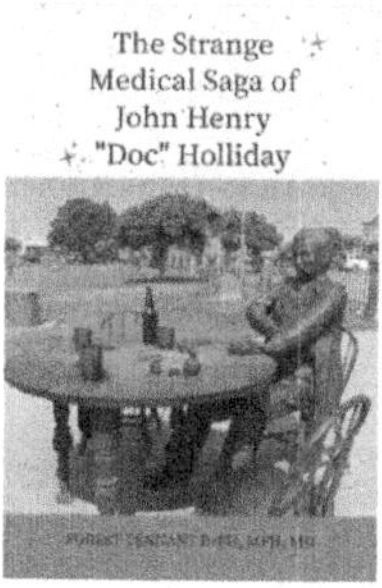


The Strange Medical Saga of "John Henry"

ISBN: 9781955934275
LOC: 2023913628

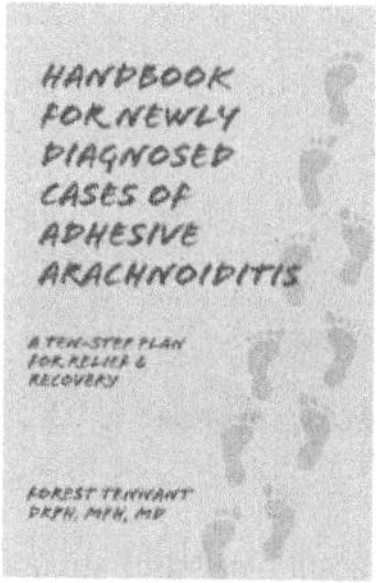


Handbook For Newly Diagnosed Cases of Adhesive Arachnoiditis

ISBN: 9781955934244
LOC: 2023908116

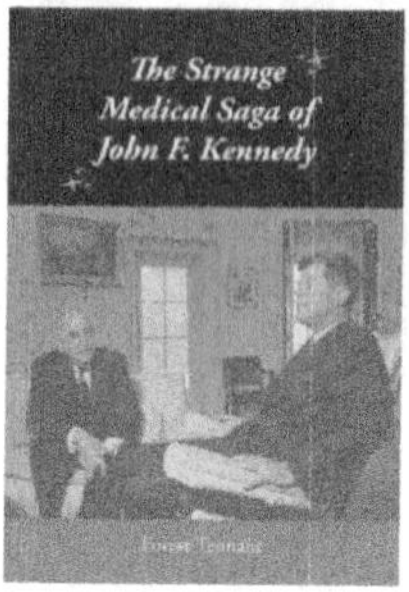


The Strange Medical Saga of JFK

ISBN: 9781955934213
LOC: 2023903440

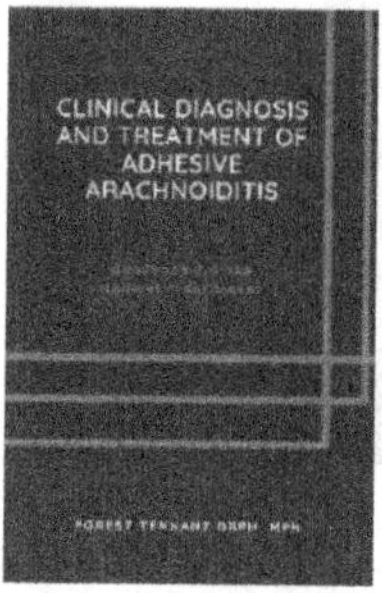


Clinical Diagnosis and Treatment of Adhesive Arachnoiditis

ISBN: 9781955934183
LOC: 2022907190

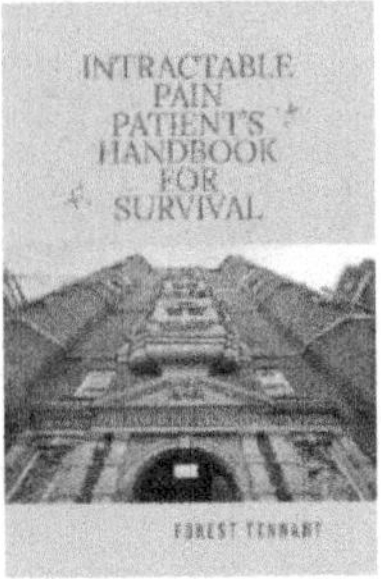


Intractable Pain Patients Handbook for Survival
ISBN: 9781955934121
LOC: 2021916464

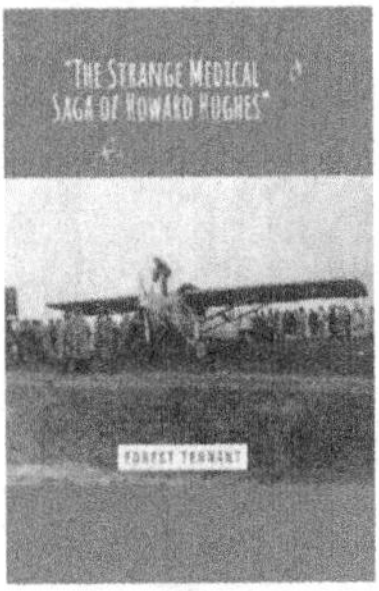


The Strange Medical Saga of Howard Hughes
ISBN: 9781955934091
LOC: 2021912855

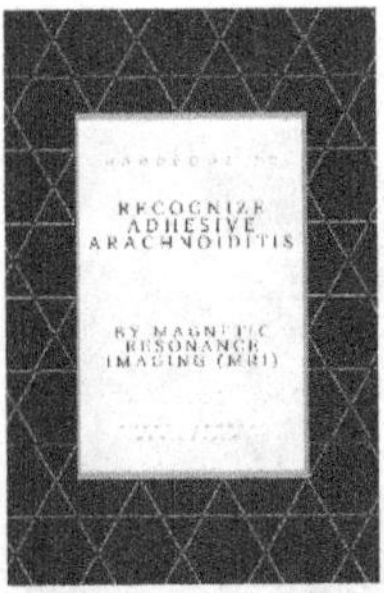


Handbook To Recognize Adhesive Arachnoiditis by Magnetic Resonance Imaging (MRI)
ISBN: 9781955934152
LOC: 2021925161

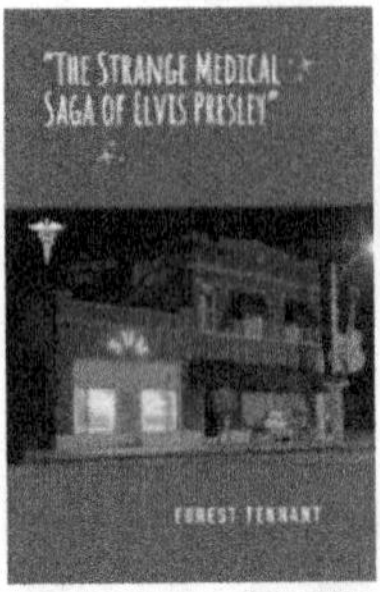


The Strange Medical Saga of Elvis

ISBN: 9781955934008
LOC: 2021911718

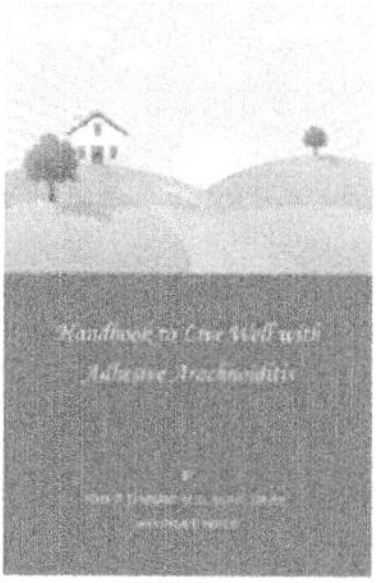

Handbook to Live Well with
Adhesive Arachnoiditis
ISBN: 978195934060
LOC: 2021912718

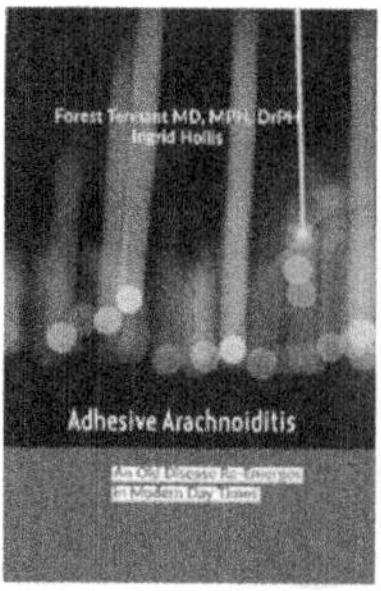


An Old Disease Re-Emerges in
Modern Times
ISBN: 9781955934039
LOC: 2021912467

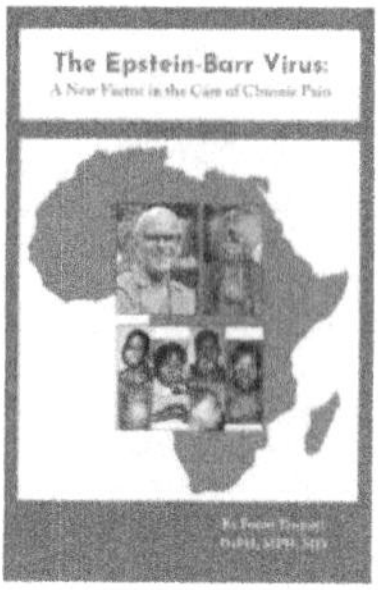


The Epstein-Barr Virus: A New
Factor in the Care of Chronic
Pain
ISBN: 9781955934428
LOC: 2024919179

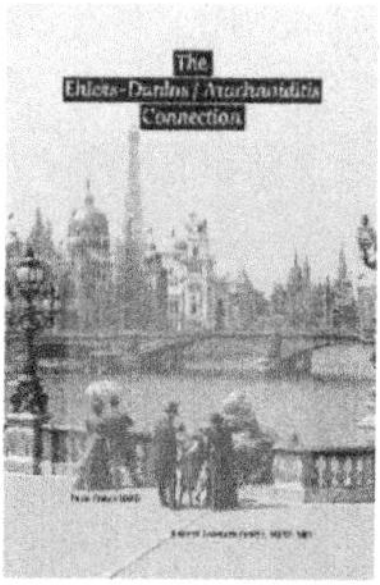

The Ehlers-Danlos /
Arachnoiditis Connection

ISBN: 9781955934381
LOC: 2024911409

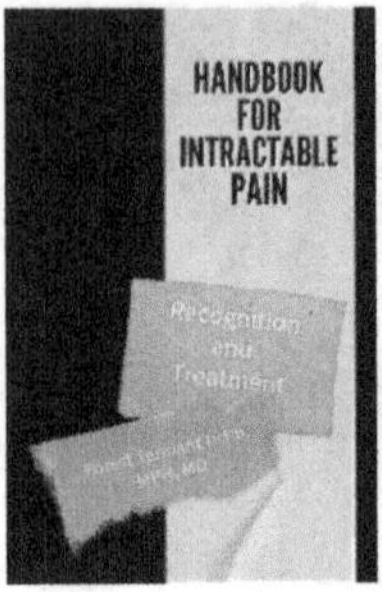


Handbook for Intractable Pain
ISBN: 9781955934329
LOC: 2023921074

Made in the USA
Monee, IL
13 September 2026

62976618R00049